# Living With

# Lupus

By

Soulja Choc

**ISBN:** 9781710581157

SCP 1st published  11/18/2019

Cover designed by:  Tina Louise  Shivers

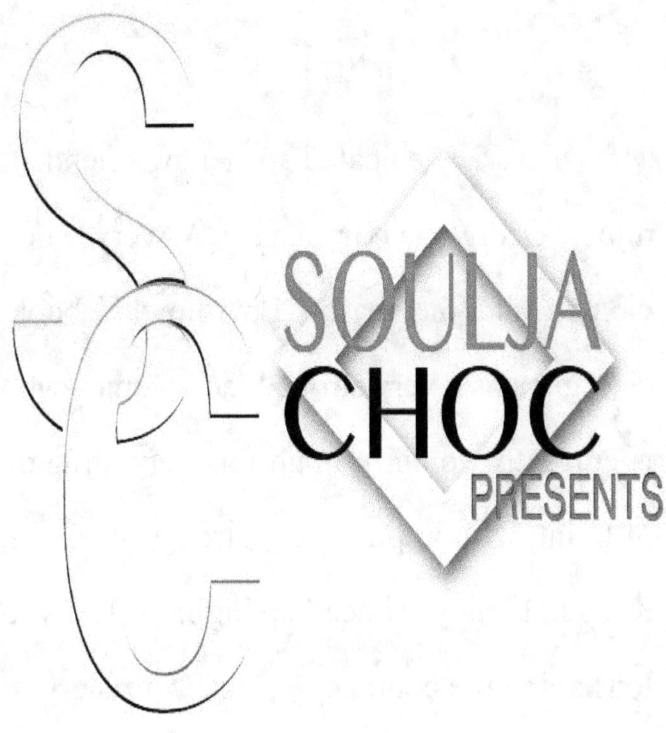

SOULJA
CHOC
PRESENTS

# Dedication

This book is dedicated to a new friend of mine, Georgiana Braham.  A very good woman and the reason I wrote this book. Georgiana is a very strong black woman who is currently going through this very struggle of living with Lupus.  Stay strong my sistah. Keep holding your head up high. I salute you for having the courage to share your story to me and the world.

# Chapter 1

## *In the Beginning*

I, Georgiana Jackson, was born and raised in Jamaica. I didn't have the best life, but my life was fair. When I was a teenager, I was fortunate enough to meet my first true love; my son. I may have been a young mother, but I was his mother. Looking into his eyes, I knew then that I had someone who would love me unconditionally. He would always be able to depend on me as well.

It was a rebirth of sorts. He brought me so much joy and happiness. It was a feeling that I never had before. I won't lie and say that being a teenage mother was easy. It most definitely was not. I did the best I could with the cards that I was dealt. Wanting better for myself and my son, I decided that some changes needed to be made.

By the age of eighteen, I left Jamaica and my son and headed to the states. I moved to Atlanta, Georgia. To say that I experienced a culture shock would be an understatement. It took many months for me to get used to the way things were done here in the States.

Don't get me wrong. I loved Jamaica. Through and through, but the states brought different opportunities for someone like me. There was so much freedom here. You weren't so controlled like back at home. Also, jobs here were plentiful. If you were willing to work, you could make it.

Schooling in the states was another huge thing. The amount of schools and programs that were offered were unbelievable. It afforded you the chance to better yourself and your job prospects as well. It was a whole new world. Literally.

I was able to find a job and begin to work. Everything was going great. Working here allowed me to pay my bills and also send money back home to Jamaica. Knowing that they were doing okay and had what they needed allowed me to sleep better at night. Much better than I had ever slept back home. It was the type of restful sleep that came when worries were lighter. A sleep I welcomed and appreciated very much.

# Chapter 2

## *Is it Love?*

I met a man after being in the states a few months. Isn't that how love always starts? Finding someone? He eventually became my boyfriend. We worked on getting to know each other for months. The more we found out about each other, the more we fell in love. It felt good, I can't deny that. To have someone who cares for you the way you care for them. Someone who wants to see you do well. Someone you can build and grow with. I was happy. We were happy.

He eventually moved in with me. It was a beautiful feeling not having to sleep alone at night any longer. Having someone who you could spend time with and not worry about where they were or who they were with. I thought I was a fairytale. But you know what they say about fairytales. They are only stories without endings.

Shortly after he moved in, I realized something that I had missed before. I don't know how I missed this red flag, but it was glowing now. My boyfriend and I had very different ideas of how our relationship roles should be. Very different.

It turned out that he thought that he could live with me and not help pay any money towards the bills. His expectations were that I work, pay the rent, bills, send money home to Jamaica, put food in the house and generally, take care of everything. As for him, well, he would get to keep his money.

He was under the mistaken assumption that this would fly with me. I didn't expect him to pay for everything or to take care of me. I could take care of myself. I had been for a long time now. However, I did expect for him to help out. If he thought he was going to be able to lay up under me and just watch me do everything, then he was sadly mistaken.

Sometimes, love is blind, but not for me. Even though I was in love with him, there was no way I was going to take care of a grown man. I already had a son back home that I was caring for.

Relationships are a two way street and he was living on a one way. The sex was great, I will give him that, but I wasn't the type of woman to allow a man to lay up and take advantage of me just because of that. There are plenty of men out there with great sex and who are willing to pay a bill or two. Knowing that, I wasn't about to be a fool for him.

Sex was important, don't get me wrong. It just wasn't something that I allowed to run my life. You can't make sound decisions if you are making them based off of how well someone lays it down in the bedroom. I refused to be ruled by lust. I had common sense and that just wasn't going to happen.

Even though it hurt, I did the only thing I could do. Told him to pack his shit and get out of my place. He thought it was a joke at first. Until I made it abundantly clear that I was serious. Once he left, I closed that door and never looked back. That was one thing about me. I never looked back. I only looked in the direction that I wanted to move. Ahead.

I knew my worth. I was a smart, beautiful, hardworking and determined woman. I decided to just live my life. Knowing that one day, the right man would appreciate those things about me. I had no plans to settle in the meanwhile. I kept on doing the things that would better me as a woman and mother. That is what was important to me. So, I pressed forward, alone.

# Chapter 3

## *CHANGES*

I had woken up early feeling good for some odd reason this morning. As I arose from the bed, I gave my joints a good stretch then headed towards the bathroom to start my morning routine. I washed my face and brushed my teeth while I waited for the water to warm up. Then, I jumped in and took a twenty-minute shower. The water felt good raining down on my body.

Once I was done in there, I got out, dried off and moisturized my skin. Then, I went into my room to pick out an outfit while my curlers heated up. I took a little extra time on my hair that morning, singing to myself the whole time. I don't know what it was, but I just felt good.

I decided that since I was up early, I would grab some breakfast. Once I was ready, looking and feeling good from head to toe, I headed out. I let the car warm up and then headed to the nearest restaurant. As I pulled into the Denny's parking lot, I got out the car and went inside. The hostess escorted me to a small booth, and I sat there all to myself.

The waiter came over to bring me my menu and I couldn't help but to notice that he was watching me intently. As if he was trying to muster up some courage. He must have, because he finally spoke.

"Please excuse me. At the risk of losing my job, I just have to say that you are on point this morning. Now, I'll give you a chance to look at the menu while I grab you a glass of water."

I smiled to myself and thought that he did look good. However, I had to remind myself that a man was not my focus. Success and a better life for me and my son was. Which urged me to look at the menu and try to ignore this handsome man that obviously had eyes for me. I will say this. If I was looking for a man right now, he would definitely get my number along with his tip.

The waiter came back and asked if I was ready to order.  And once again, I had to remind myself again that he wasn't on the menu.

"Yes. I'll take a grand slam and a glass of orange juice."

Denny's wasn't crowded that morning, so he came back with my order in no time. I ate my food and left him a five dollar tip. After I went to the front to pay for my breakfast, he met me at the door, with the five dollars in his hand.

"Pardon me. I can't accept this tip. If anything, I should be tipping you."

"Tipping me?" I asked confused.

"Yes. For looking and smelling good enough to make my entire day," he explained.

I just smiled and accepted the five dollars back. Leaving out the door, I tucked the five back in my pocket, got in my car and pulled off with that brother on my mind. He seemed like a good dude. Then again, that's how they all seem until you get to know them. As I pulled out the parking space, I looked up and saw him still watching me through the window. He winked at me. Just for the hell of it, I winked back and even blew him a kiss.

Once I drove the ten minutes to work and parked, I headed into the building, smiling. I clocked in and went to my register. I worked at Walmart. It wasn't the best job. It did, however, pay my bills and take care of my son. That was good enough for me.

Once I was settled in, my co-worker at the next register tried to get my attention.

"Hey. Psst," she said.

At first I didn't realize she was even talking to me. She kept on until I turned around.

"What girl?" I asked.

"Who is he? What's his name? Where did you meet him? I want all of the details. Now, speak," she told me.

"Girl, what are you talking about?" I asked her.

"Tell you what, on your break, go in the bathroom and look at the smile on your face. Either you met someone or I'm crazy. I mean, you always look and smell nice. But today that added with that smile and glow, it got to be a man."

"Again, I have no clue what you are talking about," I smiled.

"Well, if you just glowing like that naturally let me know your skin care routine. Cause I know I haven't felt like you look in a long time."

"Well thank you. I think," I laughed.

"I don't know. I just woke up feeling good

this morning. It was nothing more than that. I promise," I told her.

"Lies. Only more money or good dick make a woman glow like that."

Laughing, I told her that she was a fool and that there was no extra money or man anywhere around me. At least not that I knew of. Just then, a customer came to my line. I told my co-worker I would catch up with her later. I wasn't trying to get in trouble for not doing my job. That would have definitely dimmed my glow.

# Chapter 4

## *TAKING CARE OF BUSINESS*

I went back to Jamaica as often as I could to visit my son. I wanted him to know that his mother loves him and was doing this for him. Never did I want him to feel like our connection wasn't strong. Children would sometimes resent their parents when they move away to gain a better life. Not just for themselves, but the entire family. I never wanted him to feel abandoned.

Once I turned twenty-one years old, I became an official resident of the United States of America. That was what I was waiting on to bring my son back with me. Now we could be together. Things over here were different. Faster. Having going through it myself when I came over, I was able to help him. He was a fast learner as well and adapted quickly.

I still did everything I could for him to get to know his new home. Not wanting him to feel alone or out of place were good enough reasons for me. One day, while shopping at Albertson's, I could have sworn I saw the man from Denny's all that time ago.

*"Nah, Georgiana. That's crazy,"* I told myself. Except it wasn't because I never forgot a face.

When he didn't say anything, I figured that maybe I was mistaken. My son and I continued to shop. I picked out some clothes and allowed him to get some snacks that he wanted. Once we were in line, this maybe Denny's man was in the line next to me. He stepped out of line and came over to ours.

"I knew that was you," he said. "I thought I missed my opportunity that day and would never see you again," he told me.

He wasn't exactly whispering, which made us the focal point of all of the customers in line. I looked down at my son to make sure he wasn't nervous. He wasn't. He may have been the only person there not interested in our conversation.

"Yeah, I thought that was you as well. When you didn't say anything, I figured I was mistaken," I told him.

"Can I have your phone number, Instagram, or Facebook? Something. I just need to be able to contact you."

By this time, we were at the register. The cashier decided to add her two cents in.

"Girl, give him a shot. Any man willing to go through all of this and cause a scene is worth at least that," she advised me.

Then the woman behind me jumped in.

"Well, if she won't give you hers, I'll give

you mine." I cut my eyes at her to let her know to stay in her lane. I didn't need to do that though because he didn't even look in her direction. His eyes were trained on me the whole time.

I told him my name on Facebook and Instagram instead of my phone number.

"Thank you. I'll be in touch," he told me as he grabbed his basket and got back in his own line.

By the time I paid for my items and my son and I got in the car and was situated, I had a message from him.

*"Please tell me you're single?"*

*"LOL, I am. But that doesn't mean you can take me on a date. We can, however, get to know each other."*

We reached the house and went in. I put away the groceries and got my son situated. I grabbed my phone out of my purse and looked at it. I had another message from him.

*"Take your time. I'm not going anywhere. Just please, respond back."*

Smiling, I almost sent him a message. Not wanting to seem desperate, I changed my mind and decided to respond the next day. I couldn't allow him to think it was that easy to get to me. Sitting my phone down, I asked my son what he wanted to eat. Of course, he said his favorite; chili dogs.

He always said that. There was really no need to ask him. I think it might be the way I make my chili. I got pickles just big enough to give the chili that extra little kick. Then I would put a layer on the roll under the chili dog and then more on top, finishing it with a layer of ketchup. Sometimes, a line of mustard if we were feeling it.

My son helped me to set up the dinner table for us and then we sat down to eat. He then got up and helped me again to clean up. We sat on the couch and watched movies until he dozed off to sleep. I carried him to his room and put him to bed.

Then I headed into my room. I grabbed the book I was reading, "The Birth of Gutta Squad" by one of my favorite authors Soulja Choc and went back to reading until I got sleepy. It was so good, I didn't want to stop reading even when my eyelids were getting heavy. Finally, I convinced myself it would be there in the morning. After putting my book marker in to hold my page, I climbed in the bed, pulled the covers up over my head, and fell asleep.

# Chapter 5

## *FIRST DATES*

I was in my room lying across my bed reading another book; "When Hustlers and Hitmen Collide." I don't know what it was about a good urban book that I loved. It could be any number of things; the money, street wars with any number of male characters that could be book baes, or the sex. It was probably all of it.

My son knocked on my door as he stood in the doorway and I told him to come in. He knew better than to walk into my room without asking. He was a good boy.

"Come on in, baby," I told him, putting my book to the side.

"Mama, can I bring the phone to you? There is some man asking for you."

"Yes, of course," I told him.

He came in and handed me my cellphone that I had left in the living room. I guess he had decided to answer it for me. He was also protective. I was shocked to see that it was a video call. I was glad I wasn't in my silk bonnet and night clothes yet. As soon as I saw who it was, I smiled.

"I just met your son. We talked for about ten minutes. He's really smart and cool. I hope you don't mind."

My son was smiling as he walked out. Since he didn't seem agitated, I guess it was okay. It wasn't ideal. But it was okay. I needed to let him know some things though.

"It's okay. This time. I just want to let you know that I don't usually let men meet my son. Especially if they aren't going to be alone. There's no point and I don't want to confuse him. Especially if they decide to walk out," I told him.

"Well, then it's all good because I don't plan on walking out. As a matter of fact, I have an idea. Since we have a dinner date in roughly…" he said as he looked at his wrist, "Two hours, why don't you bring him with us? That way I can meet him in person. I mean the right way. Not in line at a store," he laughed. "If you feel comfortable. If not, another time. It's totally up to you."

"I think waiting is best. I just don't know you that well yet. I don't want to confuse him," I explained.

"No problem. I understand," he told me.

He noticed my facial expression and asked me what was wrong, urging me to speak my mind.

"I was just wondering, is Tyreek Myles your real name or just a Facebook alias? I guess I should have asked it before now, huh?" I added.

He laughed at me as if it was a stupid question. He then told me to hold on. He sat the phone down as I waited to see what he was doing. When he picked it back up, he had something in his hand. He held his government ID up to the phone so that I could see it.

"Here is my name."

Sure enough, it said that his name was Tyreek Myles. I smiled as he laughed at me some more.

"I always wondered it. I just didn't want to ask and seem rude."

"Listen, wanting to know who I really am is not rude. It's smart. You have to protect yourself," he told me in an understanding voice.

"You're right. I just know that people have their Facebook names in different names sometimes for many different reasons."

"Well, I have nothing to hide. Ask anything you want. I'd be happy to answer any questions you have," he assured me.

We confirmed our plans to meet at TGI Fridays in a couple of hours before hanging up. I got up off of the bed and went to my door to call my son to come to my room.

"Kevin!!"

He appeared in my doorway with a chili dog in his hand. I just shook my head back and forth.

"Hey baby. My friend said that you two talked. Is that true?" I asked.

"Yes mama. We did. Mr. Tyreek seems cool. I think he likes you," he smiled.

"Oh, he told you his name?"

"Yes. We talked for a little while. He had some questions for me. He wanted to make sure I was okay with him taking you out," he informed me.

"Questions like what?" I asked him as I walked over to my closet to pull an outfit down.

"Nothing bad. Men things mom. Geez. You should be happy he even wanted to ask me anything. Some men wouldn't do that. Then I wouldn't let you go out with them," he told me.

I looked over and realized how tall my baby was getting. He would be a man soon. I had to smile to myself. I still had questions though.

"Oh really?"

"Yes ma. See, you adults think that we kids are too young to know things. But we know things mama," Kevin said with a smile.

"Oh, do you? Things like what?"

"Mamaa…" he said before taking a bite of his food.

"Fine Kevin. If you don't want to tell me, that's fine. I just wanted to check in with you."

"It was nothing inappropriate mama or I would have hung up on him and told you," he let me know.

"That's good to know. Now, go ahead back and play your game in the living room. I need to get ready for my date," I told him.

"Okay. But not that skirt," Kevin told me as I held an outfit to my body and looked in the mirror.

"You don't like it?" I asked him.

"It's too short. Try some pants," he said on the way out the door. I laughed and went back in my closet to grab some pants.

Once I had my outfit picked out, I laid back on the bed and read three more chapters of my book. I had some time. I already showered and I needed to know what happened next. The Friday's wasn't far from my house and my hair was already done. I did, however, need to get a babysitter for Kevin. Even though he didn't think he needed one. I just wasn't ready to let him stay home alone yet.

I called my best friend Unique who didn't live too far away and asked her to come by and keep an eye on him. She said she didn't mind at all. Once I got that situated, I went ahead and began to get ready. I freshened up and sprayed my perfume, put my make-up and clothes on. By the time I was ready, Unique was knocking on the door.

"Look at you, sexy," she said.

"Girl, stop it. I was gonna wear a skirt, but I was overruled," I said to her nodding my head towards Kevin.

"Sure was…" he answered causing us both to laugh. I didn't even know he heard me. He was right; kids these days hear and know everything.

Unique came in and I told her everything she needed to know. I gave Kevin a kiss, leaving my lipstick on his face.

"Mama… dang," he complained which made Unique and I laugh more.

I left out and it took me about twenty minutes to get to the Fridays. As soon as I went to step out of the car, my phone was ringing from video chat. I answered and it was Tyreek.

"Damn, you are gorgeous," he told me.

"Boy, stop. Don't go blowing my head up," I blushed.

"I'm not. I am being serious. My very own chocolate goddess. So, I'll keep the rest of the details to myself," Tyreek told me before we hung up.

I saw him as I walked towards the door. When I got close enough, he wrapped his strong arms around me and brought me into to him. He then placed his hand, respectfully, on my lower back and escorted

me in to start our first date.

# Chapter 6

## *TWO YEARS LATER*

It has been a year since Tyreek moved in with us and everything was going great. He loved me and treated me right. He and my son, Kevin, got along really well, which was the most important thing in my book. Life was going great. Then, it changed.

I began to have back pains out of nowhere it seemed. At first, they were minor. Not enough to really bother me or cause me to need any pain medications. Being a woman, a black woman with a son at that, I did what we always do. I ignored them and kept on with life.

As time progressed the pain worsened. It got to the point where I would have to go to the hospital for them. They would run test such as X-rays and MRIs but could never find the cause. I knew I wasn't crazy. I was in pain. There was something wrong.

They would just prescribe me pain pills. They worked fine in the beginning. As time went on, they stopped working as well for the pain. To add on to that, my joints began to swell. Between that and the back pain, it was all bad. It was getting harder and harder for me to even go to work.

Even though I hung in there and kept going to work, the pain was getting to be too much. Reek and Kevin would help me as much as they could. I knew it was hard on them as well. I used to be so healthy and ready to go. Now, I was almost always in pain. Their help did manage to make things easier. It motivated me to keep going and try to push through the pain.

What I didn't understand was why the doctors couldn't find anything wrong with me. The more I went, the more they looked at me as if I was making the pain up. Like I was drug-seeking or something. I would gladly have traded them the pain pills for my health.

If it was up to me, I would never have taken

any medicine at all. I had never been one to

take medications anyway.

It was starting to upset me that people

who went to school for what seemed to be

one hundred years to learn everything there

was about bodies couldn't tell me what the

problem was with mine. Reek suggested that

I try a different doctor. At first, I didn't listen

because I had been with my doctor for years.

I figured he knew me.

When the pain continued and I wasn't

getting anywhere with him, I realized that

maybe Reek had a point. At this time, I was

willing to try almost anything. My next move

was to start looking for another doctor. I finally found one. She ran test after test on me. The same way that my last doctor did.

She still came up empty-handed. It used to cause me so much mental anguish, I would cry. Not from the pain. From the fact that no one could tell me what it was that was wrong with me. They would ask me the same questions. *"Did you sleep wrong? Did you fall?"*

How many times did I have to tell them that I didn't do anything different? I didn't sleep any different and I didn't fall. I surely would have remembered that. They may not have been able to see the back pain. How about the obvious swelling of the joints?

They could clearly see and feel that. Why couldn't they give me a reason for that? Tell me something?

The pain increased and began to affect my everyday life. When this happened, I noticed some changes in Reek. They were small at first. I didn't mention to him that I noticed it, but I did. There was nothing overt or obvious. It was in his touch and his kiss. It was… different.

I told myself that if it continued, I would bring it up. I loved him and didn't want to not be with him. However, if it continued, I would have no choice. I knew that he loved me and my son as well. My feelings were that if you loved someone and they became sick, you should stick by them. Maybe that was just me. Everyone doesn't think the same.

I didn't just have myself to consider. I had my son. I didn't want to let the small changes become so big that he would start to notice. Which, at that time, he didn't. Thank God. It was me that noticed and it hurt worse than the pains that the doctors couldn't explain.

# Chapter 7

## *MORE TEST AND A LITTLE KINDNESS*

Man, this was becoming unbearable. Here I was, on my way back to the hospital. It wasn't somewhere I wanted to be. Especially since I had just been discharged from the same place two days ago. The pain was just too much.

Yes, they had given me pills on top of pills for the pain. However, I wasn't about to overmedicate myself just because they didn't know what to do but throw pills at the problem. Hell, they didn't know what the problem was. I figured that the best thing to do was to carry my tail back to the hospital and let them continue to try and figure out what the problem was. And make no mistake, there was a damn problem.

When I arrived at the hospital, I waited for two hours, doubled over in pain before I was called to the back and given a room. As if that wasn't enough, I waited another twenty minutes for the doctor to come in and actually lay her eyes on me. At least she was nice when she finally did arrive.

"How are you doing, Georgiana? I can tell by the look on your face that you are in a lot of pain. Are the pills that I prescribed for you not working?" she asked me.

"No, they barely help at this point. To be honest, I would rather you keep the pills and find out what is wrong and fix the problem. I hate taking pills anyway."

"Well, if those pills aren't helping, I'm thinking that it may be something else wrong. Here's the plan. I'm going to send the tech on to draw some blood from you. It is going to be more blood this time. The reason for that is because I want to run some extra test. More than we did before. We need to take this approach because of the level of pain that you are having. Hopefully, when the tests come back, we will have some more answers."

Once the doctor left out, the techs and nurses descended on me. It was like everything was happening at once. They were taking my blood pressure and temperature. Then the nurse was hooking me up to monitors for my heart and goodness knows what else. The tech started to take what seemed like one a hundred vials of blood. Once they blood was taken, they started an IV. The nurse then pushed some medicine into it that took the pain away and made me doze off to sleep.

When I woke, the nurse was in the room with me. Her eyes were glued to the monitor as if she was looking for something. I asked her what it was and she told me that she was watching my vital signs. My blood pressure and heart rate more than anything.

Fine, that seemed simple enough. I felt a little better and needed to get back home to my son. I asked her when I could leave. She informed me that she didn't know quite when I would be discharged. She did know that it wouldn't be today. The doctor had already given word that I was being kept overnight for observation.

I asked the nurse to give me my phone. I needed to let Tyreek know that they were keeping me overnight. I could tell by voice that he was disappointed, but he said okay and asked if I needed anything. I didn't at the time. I called my best friend to tell her. She offered to go and get my son if I wanted her to. I thanked her and we kept on talking for about five more minutes before hanging up.

The doctor came in soon after and told me what the nurse had already explained. That she was keeping me overnight. She expected to have the results back by the time she returned to work the next morning. She assured me that she would do all she could to get to the bottom of this mystery illness. Her face and the way she said it let me know that she was serious. I appreciated it too. I thanked her with a tear dropping because I felt like she truly wanted to help me. I hadn't felt like that in awhile

She told me to just pray to God and stay positive. I agreed that I would. She then offered to have the nurses call anyone that I may have needed them to. I told her that I was fine. It was taken care of. At this point, I wasn't in pain any longer from the medicine they had given me through the IV. Heck, they could keep me for two weeks if that meant I would feel better.

I was willing to stay as long as it was going to take for them to make this problem go away. I did what she said began to pray that would be the case.

# Chapter 8

## *ANSWERS*

The next morning, the doctor came into my room to talk. She explained that she had found out why I was in so much pain. Why I was having the swelling of the joints and all of the other things that were going on. She told me that I had something called, Lupus.

It was weird. When she told me that, I was actually happy. Now that they knew what it was, I expected that they could get me on the right medications and cure me. That wasn't the case. What she told me scared me, made me upset and confused at the same time. She let me know that there was no cure for this disease.

That wasn't it either. She went on to tell me that it was also hard to treat because it mimics other diseases as well. That means that the treatment has to match with the disease that your body is mimicking at that time. She also brought me a book that would help me to better understand it. I was happy for that because this was not making any sense to me.

I read the book she gave me and it helped me to understand it a little better. In my head, I thought that Lupus was actually worse than HIV. At least with that the medicine was straight forward and helped as long as you took your medicine. It seemed that Lupus was an everyday pain and an everyday struggle.

As if that wasn't enough, this disease had the nerve to come in three different forms. *"Son-of-a-bitch..."* I thought to myself.

The first was known as Butterfly Lupus. This one was known as that because of the butterfly type pattern that it left on your skin. I mean, damn, it couldn't even let you be cute while you suffered. The next was SLE which had to do with the organs and the immune system. The last was known as medically induced Lupus. That was caused by taking certain medications over a long period of time.

I had the SLE type. Since Lupus mimics other diseases and one of my issues was the joint swelling, I was referred to a Rheumatologist. They dealt with diseases such as Rheumatoid arthritis. Which, you guessed it, makes your joints swell. That was supposed to help with my joint pain. It did help a little for the time being, that is. It was still going to be an everyday struggle.

I called home, a little more hopeful to finally know what it was that I had. To actually have a name to go with it should have been a good thing. For Tyreek and I, it wasn't. I called home and told him that they had found out what the problem was. I explained to him that I had Lupus.

I was expecting for him to be supportive. The opposite was true. He let me know in no uncertain terms that he didn't want anything to do with me and this disease. He said that it was too much for him and he didn't want to be around it. He was acting like I had AIDS or something that he could catch. He didn't even attempt to understand it. He just wanted out.

One thing I didn't have time for was trying to comfort him and worry about what he was going through. I had enough on my plate with this everyday battle. I let him know that since he didn't want to be around it or me, he could pack his things and be gone by the time I got back home…

My son was staying with Unique. I called her and let her know that she could bring Kevin to me. She offered to keep him longer. I told her that it was fine. I needed him home so that I could explain to him what was going on. I also needed to prepare him to go with his father. I didn't want him to see me going through all of the different pain and treatments. It was a lot for a child. Hell, it was a lot for me.

My baby didn't want to leave me. He wanted to stay and help me. Watch over me and make sure that I was alright. I loved him even more for that. The unconditional love that he brought into this world with him for me was showing. Just knowing that I had him made me want to fight harder. And so I did.

# Chapter 9

## *WHAT'S BEST FOR HIM*

I was finally home from the hospital after all of that time. Being back with my son was my goal and now we were back together, I was actually feeling amazing. Well, there was still some pain, but it was nothing like it had been before.

I took that time to spend time with my son. We played games, talked and read books. I even felt good enough to cook for him that night. I would lay in his bed with him and we read together before he went to sleep. Then I tucked him in.

After he was asleep, I just stood in the doorway and watched him for a while. I had missed all of this. At this point, I was doing anything to be near him. I had missed him so much. Even though he was getting older, he allowed me to baby him a little bit. I appreciated that.

Once I was finally able to pull myself away from him, it was time for me to go to bed next. I went into my room, got undressed and climbed in between the sheets. It felt so good to be back in my own bed and not in a hospital. Grabbing my remote, I turned the TV on and watched it until I fell asleep.

I woke up the next morning and hopped in my shower. Once I was done, I stood there and looked at myself in the mirror and smiled. I was still feeling better. Not waking up in the amount of pain that I had been in felt great. I brushed my teeth and got dressed. Once I was together, I headed into the kitchen and made breakfast for the two of us.

After the food was done, I woke my son up and sent him into the bathroom to wash his face and brush his teeth so that we could eat together. Once we were done eating, I washed the dishes as he went into the living room and watched cartoons. When I finished cleaning the kitchen, I headed in there to join him on the couch.

Kevin snuggled up under me and I let him. Then, he began to talk.

"Mom, why are you always in the hospital? I miss you when you're gone. I mean, auntie Unique is fun and everything and she treats me real nice. I just miss you. That's all."

Hearing him say that broke my heart. I missed him when I was gone, too. I hated that I always had to be away from him now. He went on. "I just like it when we sit up and read together before bed. Stuff like that."

"I know, baby. Believe me, it's not what I want. I go to the hospital so that they can work on making me feel better. That way I can do more things for you. That's why I'm going to be sending you to stay with your father for a while. The doctors have a few more things to do before I can feel better more often. After that, I won't be in the hospital as much. Then we can spend more time together. Like we used to," I explained.

The problem with the explanation is that it was half the truth and half a lie. I was sending him to his father. However, I had no clue how long it would be to get me to feeling better more often. Especially since this disease didn't have a cure. I prayed it wouldn't be long though. Maybe we could figure out some treatment that kept me feeling this good. Or even better. Then he could be back with me. Where he belonged.

Once we were done speaking about it, I left Kevin to watching his cartoons and headed into my bedroom. I called his father and asked him if he would be willing to fly over and pick our son up if I paid for the flight. He told me that he would be happy to. Then he asked when I wanted him to come. I explained that as soon as possible would be good. Today even. Knowing that it was short notice.

He agreed. If I paid for it, he would prepare to come now. After we hung up, I made the travel arrangements for his father to come over and for the two of them to go back together. Next, while I was still not in too much pain, I called my son into my room and told him to get dressed. We were going somewhere fun.

After we were both ready, we headed out and I took him to Chuck E Cheese. He played for a couple of hours and we even took pictures. I needed something to remember this day by. The rest, I would send with him for the same reason. We exchanged our tickets for prizes on the way out.

Neither one of us was in the mood for pizza, so we didn't eat at Chuck E Cheese's. Instead, we stopped at Denny's and got some food. From there, we went to Walmart. There were a few items I needed to get for him for his trip back with his father. Also, some snacks, knick-knacks, brand new pair of pajamas and some other things that I thought he might want to have.

When we got back home, Kevin went into his room and laid down to take a nap. I went into the living room and as soon as I laid on the couch, I was sleep as well. I woke from my nap and found him standing there, watching me.

"What is it, baby?" I asked him.

"Mom, can we watch a movie?" he asked.

"Yes, sure. Which one do you want to put in?" I asked him.

"Lion King," Kevin answered. It was one of his favorites. Mine as well. We put it in and started to watch it.

He must have really tired himself out today because he fell back asleep during the movie. I got him up and walked him into his room. We got his clothes off and pajamas on. I grabbed the book we were reading together and by chapter two, he was back asleep. I kissed his forehead, pulled the covers up around him and left out.

I was beat myself. Once I got undressed, I climbed in bed as well. As soon as my head hit the pillow, I was sleeping, too.

The next evening his father arrived to pick him up and take him back with him. We spent a little time at the house together. Catching up and whatnot. Then he took us out to dinner. He wanted to spend a little family time together for our son. That way he could see that we were all on the same page.

We went back by the house, picked up my son's packed bags and I dropped them off at the airport. By the time I got back home, the pains were really beginning to kick back in. Well, if they were going to come, this was the time. I was just glad that my body had waited for my son to be safely with his father before they kicked up again.

I called Unique and she came right over to get me and take me to the hospital. On the way there, Unique asked me if I was going to miss my son. I actually began to cry because I already missed him. The right decision had been made though. I knew that.

I couldn't afford to keep him with me with all of this back and forth going on with my health. I know that Unique said she didn't mind caring for him and me. It wasn't that I didn't trust her or appreciate the offer. It was that I didn't think that it was fair to her to keep pawning him off on her. Especially when this disease was so unpredictable.

Once I arrived at the hospital, Unique stayed with me until I was checked into a room. She waited about thirty more minutes to make sure that I was alright, then let me know to contact her if I needed anything. I thanked her again before she left.

The doctor asked me what exactly it was that was hurting. I told him and they ran more test. When he came into the room next, his announcement threw me for a loop. He told me that I was going to be having heart surgery the next day. He suggested that I call anyone I needed to and let them know that.

Unique was the only one for me to call. She told me she was praying for me and would be there in the morning. They actually wanted to do the surgery that day. The only reason they didn't was because I was in the midst of a flare-up. When that happens it takes longer to heal.

I was so used to being in the hospital, it was a shame. Still, I didn't like it. Whenever I was admitted, I never spent less than two days. It could take over a week to get everything under control so I could return home. It was still depressing.

The next morning they woke me up to get me prepared for surgery. The doctor came in to check on me and asked how I was feeling. I told him it was about the same. He informed me that my Lupus was still flaring up. He couldn't wait for it to subside though. He had to go on with the surgery.

As I was readied, I began to overthink. What if something happened? This was my heart they were going to be working on. I needed that right? I grabbed my phone and called my son's father. I told him what was going on. Then, I made him promise that if anything happened to me, he would raise our son and make sure that he knew how much I loved him. That he would never let him forget me either.

After I made him promise, he tried to comfort me by telling me that I would be fine. I was strong and this surgery would go the way it should go. I appreciated that. Once I was off the phone with him, my next call was to God. I had questions. Even though I know that you aren't supposed to question him; I needed to know. Why me? What had I done to deserve this disease?

I had done all I could to be a good woman, a good person, and a good mother. Why do these things always happen to the good people? No answer was forthcoming. Even then I kept the faith. I would continue to pray for healing of my body. I truly believed that one day, by his grace and mercy, I would -wake up Lupus free. I had to believe that.

They took me back to the operating room and put me to sleep. After they completed the surgery, I woke up in recovery room. The doctor came in and told me that everything went great. Once I healed up, everything would be fine.

That was great to hear. I went back to praying to God that I would heal. Not just from this surgery, but from this disease. I thought about everything. Especially being there for my son. I knew that I didn't have any control. It was in God's hands. He finally spoke back to me. It wasn't in words. It was in a feeling.

This feeling of peace came over me. It told me that I was here on this earth for a purpose. It hadn't yet been accomplished, so I wasn't going anywhere yet. I turned my mind to positive thoughts. Thoughts of healing and getting everything back in order so that I could bring my son back for good. This back and forth wasn't good for him.

I knew that he wanted to be with me as much as I wanted him here. It made me want to heal all the more. He gave me the strength not to give up, and so I continued to fight.

# Chapter 10

### THE INCIDENT

### Three months later

My son was visiting me for a week and today was his last day here. I had the whole day mapped out for us. We would have breakfast. From there, he would get a haircut at the barbershop. Then we would go and see a movie together. It was a lot to squeeze in, but he was leaving in the morning.

I wanted to do as much as I could with him while I wasn't in pain and he was all mine. The first five days he was visiting me, I could barely get out of the bed the pain was so bad. All we did was stay in the house. He helped me as much as he could. He was more understanding than other people I had met.

The day before, the pain had let up some and we headed to the park. Now, I was feeling excellent so we took advantage of that. He ordered our favorite from our favorite restaurant; a grand slam from Denny's. We sat at the table and just spent time together and enjoyed the food.

I could tell that Kevin didn't want to leave me and go back home with his father.

He was trying to be strong and I could tell. It wasn't that he didn't love his father. He did. It was that he loved and felt protective over me. I could appreciate his mixed feelings and the fact that he wanted to care for me. But, it was my job to do what was best for him. No matter how much it tore me up.

After finishing up our food, we left Denny's. The next stop was the barbershop to make sure Kevin was looking good before he headed back to be with his father. We waited twenty minutes for his turn in the chair. Once Kevin was situated and the barber started, I leafed through a magazine pretending not to be paying attention to the barbershop gossip.

I was though. I couldn't help it. They weren't exactly whispering.

I thought to myself that men talked about women gossiping. But it seemed to me that they were running their mouths in here more than we ever did. Especially in the hair salon. They had us beat by a long shot. I just smirked to myself at the irony in that.

Once the barber was done, he called me up to make sure that I was satisfied. I was. It was a sharp cut and line up. As I reached in my purse for the money to pay, in walked my ex. He loudly started to embarrass me by calling out to the barber.

"HEY, RON! You better get away from her. She got that shit!" he screamed across the barbershop.

I couldn't believe my eyes or my ears. He was staring at me as if I had AIDS or something. I looked around and all eyes were definitely on me. I wanted to disappear. Instead, I checked his ignorance.

"First of all, I don't have '*that shit*' or whatever you want to call it. I have Lupus. That's an illness. And there is no one in here that could possibly get it by being near me, touching me, or having sex with me. So, the next time you want to tell somebody business, make sure that you have your facts straight. That's what's wrong with black men these days. Always trying to put a sister down. Half of the time don't even know what you talking about. It's not like I had sex with the wrong person. I mean, unless I count you. This disease came on out of nowhere. It could even happen to your mama. What if it was your mama? Would you want someone screaming some ignorant shit across the supermarket at her?" I asked him.

He stood there looking confused as hell. He looked like he wanted to say something. Before he could fix his lips to get it out, people began to talk.

"Daaang… she told him," one person muttered.

"Yeah. He must be slow. He don't even know what Lupus is," another young woman stated.

Then Ron looked over to him and checked him as a real man should.

"Look my man, you can't come in here disrespecting my clients. If you can't understand that, just don't come up in here," he told him.

"It's like that?" he asked Ron.

"Hell yeah, it's like that. You come up in here trying to embarrass this queen like that. She ain't say or do nothing to you. That shit wasn't even cool," Ron replied.

"I feel you," my ex said looking embarrassed and still thrown for a loop. "I'll get with you another time."

Ron just nodded his head to let him know that he was disappointed in him. When I tried to pay for the haircut, Ron wouldn't accept the money. He told me that the haircut was on the house. I still tried to pay him and he continued to refuse.

As I walked away, he stopped me by the door and spoke.

"I liked the way you handled yourself with class. I appreciate if you wouldn't allow his bad manners to stop you from coming back here."

"No, I wouldn't do that, Ron. I appreciate you stepping in as well. It's just that my son doesn't live out here any longer. But whenever he comes to visit and needs a haircut, we will be here. It's not your fault that he's an idiot," I assured him.

"I know. I just feel bad because this is my place of business."

We left the barbershop and headed to the movies. We didn't talk about what happened. I was fine with that. We watched Gemini man. That was a good movie. It was smooth how they cloned him. Once the movie was over, we headed home and talked until we were both tired. He went to his room to lie down and I did the same.

# Chapter 11

## *ANOTHER SURGERY*

The next morning, we both overslept. Kevin had to rush to shower so that I could get him to the airport in time. I made sure all his things were ready. I went out front to warm the car up. He was coming out of his bathroom as I was headed into mine.

I used the restroom, washed my face and brushed my teeth as he put his clothes on. We left and had a few minutes to spare since we moved so quickly earlier. I stopped at McDonald's to get him something to eat before he got on the plane. We ate in the car.

Once we arrived at the airport, I parked and then walked him in. Kevin was flying as an unaccompanied minor so I had to make sure that he was checked in correctly and given to the right staff member. I stayed with him until they called for him to board. As I was walking back to the car, pain started to creep back in.

I was happy that my son was gone. I was sick and tired of this pain shit. It seemed to come on from out of nowhere. I tried to hurry back to the house to lie in the bed and get some rest. Take some medicine and hoped that helped as well. I tried to get home as fast as I could. I hated driving when I was in pain. It was dangerous.

After making it home safely, I ran some hot bath water and prayed that it would make the pain go away. It didn't. I wasn't home a full hour before I had to call an ambulance to come and get me. Fifteen minutes later, they arrived and I was being loaded onto a gurney for the ride to the hospital. As they drove me to the hospital, I was asking the Lord why me. What had I done to deserve this? I was a good woman with a good heart. Why did I have to suffer like this?

I was just searching for an answer from God for those questions. It didn't come. We finally arrived at the hospital and I was checked in. They called my doctor and she asked them to put me on the phone. When I was handed the receiver, she told me that she was having me transferred to the hospital where she was working that week and had privileges. It was also a heart center.

Once I was transported there, she gave me medicine to help with the pain while they ran tests. After the tests came in, she informed me that I would have to have another surgery. Also on my heart. The cardiologist would be putting stents in to keep the pathways open and the blood flowing. Basically saving my life. This would mark heart surgery number two.

One thing that I really appreciated about my doctor was that she always tried to be understanding and make things as bearable as they could be. Especially since she and I knew that this wouldn't stop the pain completely. If we knew anything, these symptoms and others, would come back.

My doctor left and I tried to watch TV. My eyes were getting heavy. I was exhausted. That mixed with the medicine that they had been giving me were not helping me stay awake either. I continued to watch TV until I felt myself fading into sleep. I said a prayer that all went well with the surgery the next

day and then gave in to the exhaustion.

# Chapter 12

## *SOMEONE TO TRUST*

I was recovering from my second surgery. All I could think to myself was, "I hate this shit." When you are sick and in constant need of medical attention, all types of thoughts go through your mind. This surgery was for my heart to place stents.

The doctors informed me that I should heal faster this time. The reason being that I wasn't having a flare-up right now. Healing from my first heart surgery was hell due to that exact thing. I just wanted to pain to be over already. The truth is, there is no cure for this. I would be dealing with this on some level for the rest of my life.

I don't know. Sometimes I think to myself that if I only had a good man to be by my side and support me through this, I might do a little better. It would make everything easier. As of right now, I hadn't met the right one. I wasn't interested in just being a piece of ass. I wanted love and commitment.

It wasn't because men didn't approach me. They did. When I was well enough to be out and about, the men did try their hands. I knew within the first minute if I was interested in allowing them to take me out on a date or not. They had to be a certain type of man for me to even give them a chance.

I needed a man that I could depend on. I didn't have time to waste. With this illness, I needed someone that I could trust fully. Lupus can sometimes render you paralyzed. During the times when your joints lock up, you literally can't move. That makes you vulnerable to anyone that doesn't have your best interest at heart.

If you aren't around family or friends when that happens, someone with ill-intentions could take advantage of you when you are in a state like that. That is why I can't let just any man into my life. I would pray that something like that would never happen to myself or others in my situation. However, people these days are sick themselves. It's just in their head. They would take advantage of a person who they were supposed to be loving and caring for with no remorse. No, I wasn't looking for that.

Another problem with having Lupus is that you can't always see the pain coming. The pain comes with the flare-ups. It can just hit unexpectedly. You can be having a great day, going on about your business and then have an onset, turning your great day into a bad one to say the least.

I was at home now on bedrest. Even being on bedrest, I was happy not to be in the hospital. I hated being there. Even though I knew it was par for the course. I knew that there were times that I needed that extra help and attention from the doctors and nurses. Which is why I had to be admitted so often. Still, there was no place like home.

Unique was coming over to visit me. She had let me know that she would be there in about half an hour. I heard the doorbell ring and it was her. I knew I wasn't supposed to be moving around but the door wasn't going to answer itself. When I opened it, there she stood. She had two bags in her hand. One held books and the other had donuts.

That was what I loved about my best friend. She was so thoughtful. And besides that, she knew me so well. Well enough to show up with donuts. She was always trying to keep me upbeat and happy. Taking care of the things I needed and making sure I was happy. She was more than a friend. She was a sister.

We went in and sat on the couch and talked. After a while, she pulled the books out and showed them to me. She knew my taste in books as well. Having picked up an urban series called, "In Love With a Cali Hood Boss." It was a six book series and I could not wait to start reading it. The cover alone let me know that this was about to be a great read.

Next, we began to work on the donuts she had brought. Unique grabbed the remote and started looking for movies. She found one of my favorite movies on the firestick, Poetic Justice. We watched it together. When it was over, she stood and got ready to leave. Hugging me and letting me know that if I needed anything, no matter the time, to let her know. I promised that I would. I didn't know what I would do without her. I appreciated her consistency. She kept my spirits up. Yes, a sister. That's what she was.

# Chapter 13

## *THE FIGHT CONTINUES*

I was at home in the middle of a flare-up. The doctor had once again put me on bedrest. This time, it was for the swelling around my spine. I wouldn't wish this on my worst enemy. I had been doing well for a few days. Then it hit again. It was a never-ending cycle.

Having to depend on other people was new to me and not something that I wanted to get used to. This diagnosis was forcing my hand in that department. And I hated it. I was so independent and active before this. Now, I damn near had to plan my life around this shit. Who wants to live like this? No one in their right minds.

Since my diagnosis, I have had more than one heart surgery and a brain tumor that had to be removed. Now, I was having issues with my eyesight. It was touching me in every part of my life and body. All I could do was continue to pray that the doctors would one day find a cure. I know that was a long way off. Hell, I would take something that would at least help with the pain.

Then at least all of us that suffered with this horrible illness could go about our lives with some normality and peace.  Hell, I would take a half ass normal life at this point. I knew that they were trying. Doctors and scientist all over the world were working together to try and find a cure. I knew it was coming, just wished it would come a little faster. It's hard to be patient when in these shoes.

All of the types of Lupus are bad. Some are worse than others. Sometimes, I dream about waking up and not having Lupus any longer. I am carefree, playing with my son. We go out for walks and chili dogs. There is no pain and no worry about the next flare-up. When I wake up and realize it was just a dream, I get so upset I could cry. That's where my love of books really saves me. It provides an escape from my reality. The imagination and words that these authors use to describe their stories sweep you up in the story. The different plots and characters sometimes dull the pain more than the medicine.

As a booklover, I experiment with different authors and genres. I love giving new authors a chance. Unique and I have our own little book club. We will sit side by side and read. Yes, reading, praying and holding out hope that I will find someone to look past the Lupus and see me for the good and loving woman that I am are my coping strategies. That's what keeps me grounded and moving forward. Even when I want to quit. I know for the sake of my son, I never will. So, I continue to fight on team "Fuck Lupus" until one day, they find the cure.

*Words from the Author and advice from
Georgiana*

I decided to write this book because a friend of mine, Georgiana, is struggling with this disease right now. Having no clue about this disease, I had to rely on her to explain it to me. This is her story about her struggle. I wanted to help bring awareness to this terrible disease. There is someone out there who may have it or know someone with it who needs to know they are not alone.

I asked Georgiana what advice she would have for someone who has just been diagnosed with Lupus. Her response was *"My best advice is to take care of yourself. Do what helps you deal with your situation best. There is no one size fits all to coping with this. Lastly, find yourself a great and dependable support team. That makes all the difference.*"-Georgiana

AVAILABLE     ON

AMAZON.COM

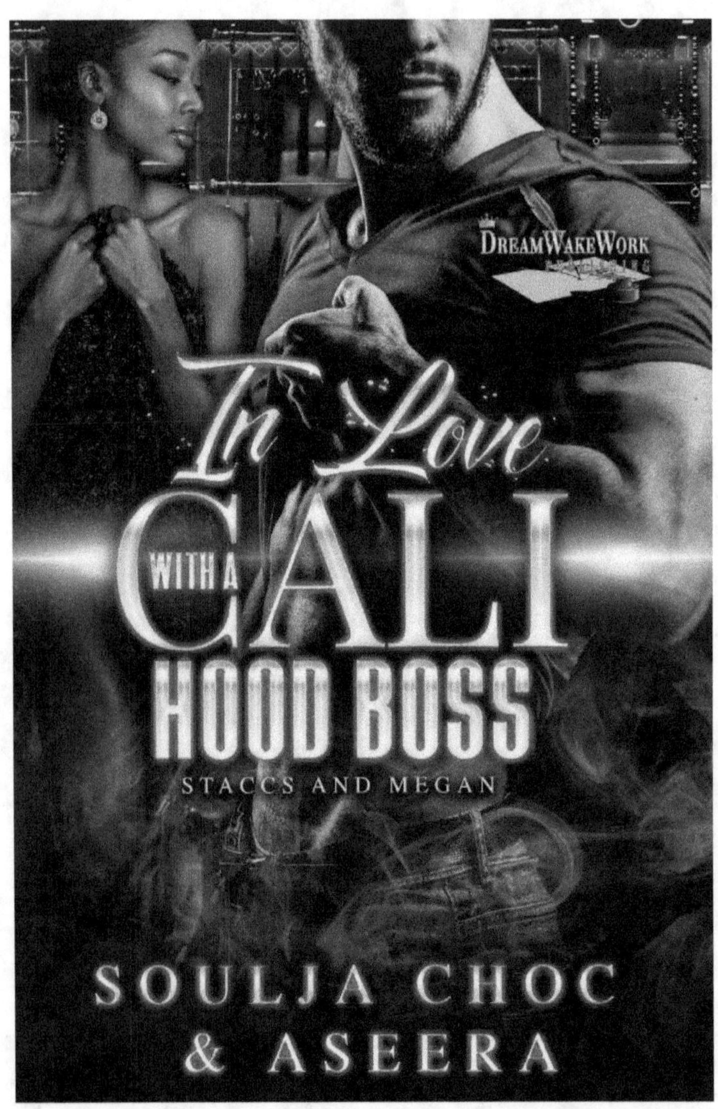


Completed Series

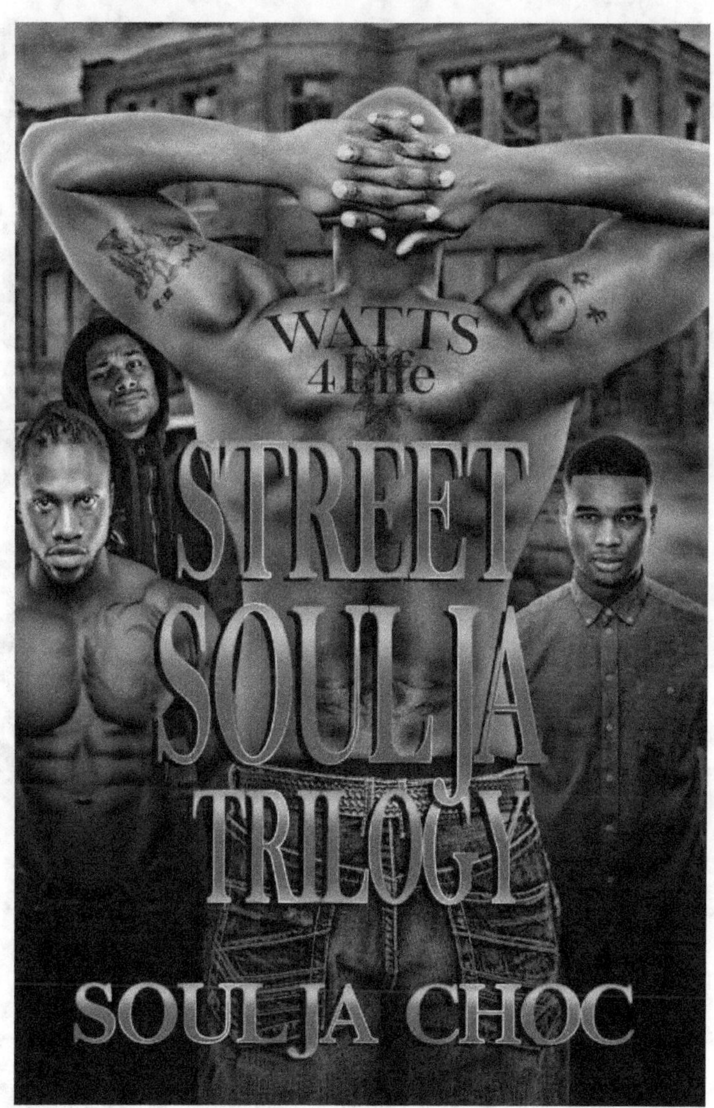

WATTS
4 Life
STREET
SOULJA
TRILOGY
SOULJA CHOC

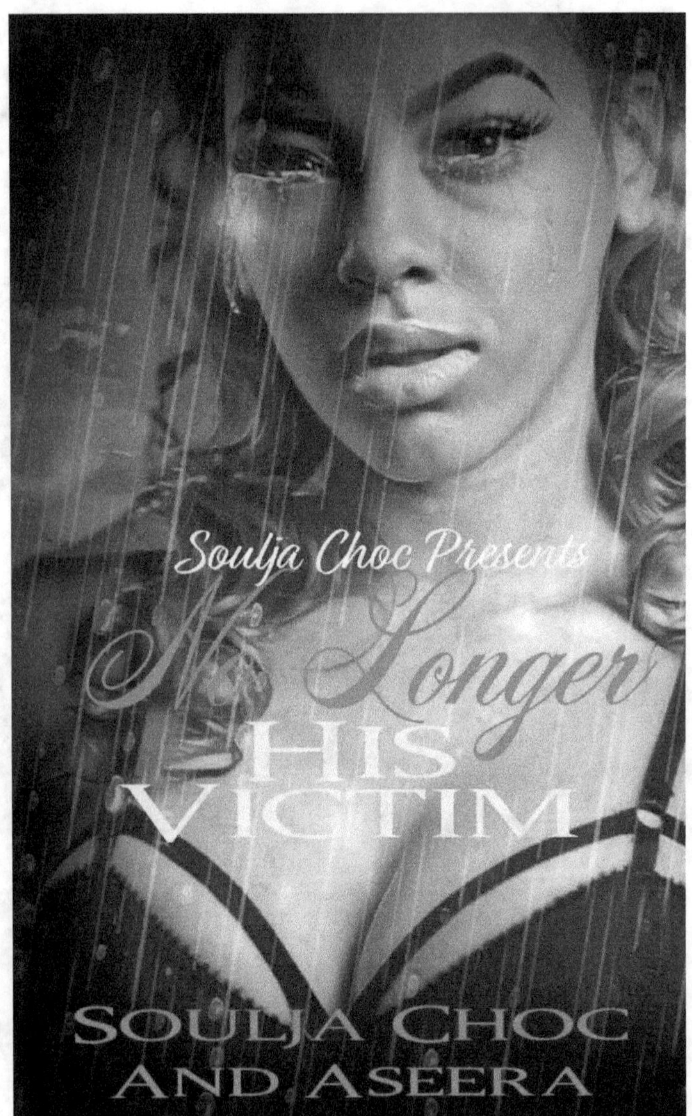

Soulja Choc Presents
No Longer
HIS
VICTIM
SOULJA CHOC
AND ASEERA

SOULJA CHOC PRESENTS
BORN
TO BE
KING
BEST SELLING AUTHOR
SOULJA CHOC